DEDICATION

I dedicate this book to my family. Thank you for always telling me that I'm the greatest cook in the entire galaxy.

TABLE OF CONTENTS

Beyond the Diet with Healthy Diet Recipes

An Easy Guide to a Healthy Lifestyle

By: Anna Reed

9781634289702

PUBLISHERS NOTES

Disclaimer – Speedy Publishing LLC

This publication is intended to provide helpful and informative material. It is not intended to diagnose, treat, cure, or prevent any health problem or condition, nor is intended to replace the advice of a physician. No action should be taken solely on the contents of this book. Always consult your physician or qualified health-care professional on any matters regarding your health and before adopting any suggestions in this book or drawing inferences from it.

The author and publisher specifically disclaim all responsibility for any liability, loss or risk, personal or otherwise, which is incurred as a consequence, directly or indirectly, from the use or application of any contents of this book.

Any and all product names referenced within this book are the trademarks of their respective owners. None of these owners have sponsored, authorized, endorsed, or approved this book.

Always read all information provided by the manufacturers' product labels before using their products. The author and publisher are not responsible for claims made by manufacturers.

This book was originally printed before 2014. This is an adapted reprint by Speedy Publishing LLC with newly updated content designed to help readers with much more accurate and timely information and data.

Speedy Publishing LLC

40 E Main Street, Newark, Delaware, 19711

Contact Us: 1-888-248-4521

Website: http://www.speedypublishing.co

REPRINTED Paperback Edition: ISBN: 9781634289702

Manufactured in the United States of America

Chapter 1- Gained Weight? Go for Healthy Diet

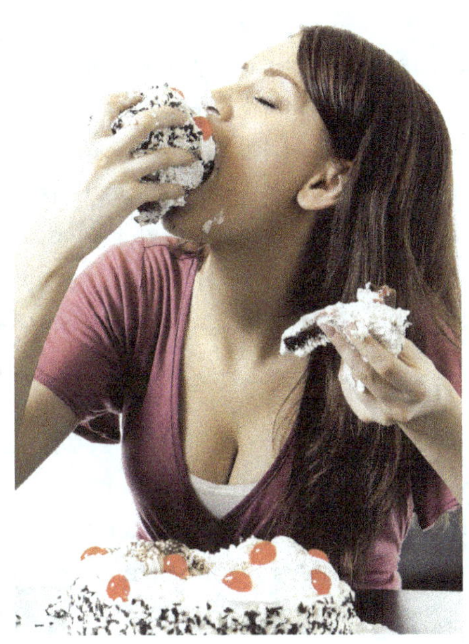

With the rush of our everyday lives, the advancement of technology, along with the conveniences of fast food, it sure is hard to stay active and eat a healthy, balanced diet. But if you know how to do it, it can be done, even with a busy lifestyle.

In this first section of the book we are going to look at:

• All the reasons why we gain weight,

• The people we need to talk to when we decide we are ready to lose the weight,

• Why keeping yourself on a schedule actually helps you to lose the weight,

• Weight loss secrets,

• Plus many other subjects that will help you to learn how to finally take the weight off and keep it off once and for all

The Major Causes of Weight Gain

We eat more calories than our body needs in a day, so the excess gets stored as fat. Our human bodies are designed in such a way that when in times it was harder to get food, our bodies could be prepared by having stored extra calories in times of plenty in the form of fat. Now, with the ease with which we get food, a lot of people tend to overeat, and this is a severe problem that causes a huge number of people to become overweight or obese.

• Genetics play a factor as well by setting basic parameters on the metabolic efficiency of your body. People who are overweight many times have very efficient metabolisms, meaning their body needs less calories per day than others to operate, and they store the excess calories as fat. Also you have a greater risk of being obese if one of your parents is and an even greater risk if both parents are.

• Your metabolic rate. Besides genetics, your metabolic rate depends on how active you are. It is said that every ten years past our mid-twenties we lose about 10% of our metabolic rate. This probably does not have to do completely with age, however, but instead with how active we are. The more active we are, the more muscle mass we can retain, or even build, and in turn the more fit we are because muscle tissue is metabolically active whereas fat is not. On the other hand, if we lead a basically sedentary life, we are much more likely to be able to gain weight as we lose muscle mass.

• Eating patterns. People's eating habits make a huge difference in determining their weight. When foods high in fat or sugars are favored, this of course can cause much weight gain. Also, how you serve the food, i.e. do you put the portions on everyone's plate or do you bring it all to the table and serve it the food family style where everyone can take as much as they want? Portion size is one of the main reasons people eat too much. Also, how have you learned to eat? If you are a fast eater, you may not even realize the cues your stomach gives you that it is full.

• Larger portion sizes. Over time, larger portions of food have become the norm, especially at many restaurants. Weight has also gone up because of this.

• Exercise or the lack thereof. Exercise is essential to a healthy lifestyle and to maintaining a healthy weight. When you exercise, especially when you include strength training in your workouts, you gain muscle mass and raise your metabolism and in turn the muscle helps to burn more fat. In turn, you will weigh less and you will look leaner and firmer because muscle takes up less space than fat. Plus, strength training helps reduce the risk of accidental injury, improves your bone density, helps with digestion and helps in lowering your blood pressure, cholesterol and triglyceride levels.

As you can see, even if your genes make it easier to gain weight than other people, diet and exercise are the two main factors that affect your health and weight. Regular exercise is essential to getting to and maintaining a healthy weight – and so is what you eat, how you eat and how much you eat.

Learn portion control. This is usually a huge factor for most people, and they do not realize how much they are actually eating. A portion of food the size of your fist is generally all that should be eaten at one time, because that is the size of your stomach as well.

Eating several small meals a day, rather than two or three big ones, will help you to be able to eat less and also not be hungry in the early days of forming this habit. Another vitally important thing is to never skip breakfast, as these sets up your metabolism for the day. If you don't eat breakfast, your body will go into defense mode and store more fat because it will think you are starving.

Try slowing down your eating as well if you have the habit of eating fast. This way you can feel the signals from your stomach when you have had enough, before you stuff yourself full. When you have done that, you know for sure you have eaten too much. In reality, on a scale of 1-10 of fullness, we should feel right in the middle, around a 5, when we are done eating. It takes some practice, but you can learn this trick and you will feel so much better knowing you did not stuff yourself to the maximum capacity.

Another thing to watch of course is your intake of fatty and sugary foods. We all need nutrients, including healthy fats, to keep us balanced, but eating a lot of junk food and sugary drinks will attribute greatly to us gaining more weight. Processed foods don't generally have a lot of nutrients in them, or any at all, and they are high in salt, sugar, and unhealthy fats.

In today's busy lifestyles, we may not realize how often we are eating these foods. If you are one who is always ordering out for work, or going out to dinner as well, this is not going to keep you healthy because you do not have the control as to what is being put in your food (except special ordering at a restaurant) and it is much harder to make sure you are eating the right kinds of things and getting all of your nutrients. Going out to eat is fine every once in a while, but be sensible in what you are choosing, and you don't have to clear your plate of the large servings you will most likely be given.

Should I Go On A Diet?

When most people think of losing weight, they think of going on a diet. Many times, this means finding some fad diet that is probably popular at the current time, and trying to follow all of its crazy rules and recipes, like lemon juice, cayenne pepper and maple syrup. But honestly, who enjoys these things? Do you like cutting out entire food groups such as carbohydrates or drinking crazy concoctions that simply do not taste very good and do not fill you up?

It is doubtful that anyone does. Yes, there are other diet plans out there that have a lot of merit to them, and if a diet is the way you want to go, then researching the different ones out there is very advisable so that you can find a reasonable, sensible diet plan that is not going to harm you or make you go crazy with hunger, causing you to fail in the end anyway.

Choosing the Right Diet Plan

When you are ready to choose your diet or eating plan, there are certain things that you must take into consideration to make sure that you are picking one that will help you to attain the weight loss goals you have and to make sure you are staying healthy. Some diets, as we mentioned, do not contain the right balance of nutrition that your body's needs, and can therefore make you sick, and won't help you to lose weight properly.

Here are some important things to keep in mind when choosing the right diet plan:

• Realistic Expectations: You must realize that losing weight is a process and takes time. The length of time to achieve your goals depends on how much you have to lose to bet to your goal weight. You do not want to take on a crash diet plan that promises you to lose a lot of weight in a short amount of time, as that will most likely be a very unhealthy and an unsafe option for you. After the initial two or three weeks when weight loss is rapid because of water loss, after that you should be losing around 1-2 pounds a week to maintain healthy weight loss.

• The Right Nutrition: Make sure you look over any diet plans you are considering thoroughly and see what they allow or suggest for you to eat. If it has a balanced-looking diet to it with the right amounts of foods from the main food groups, you are probably looking at a plan that is safe. Any of the fad diets that cut out whole food groups, or make you starve yourself or drink strange concoctions are not safe. You also want the right amount of protein, carbohydrates, fiber and make sure you are getting no more than 30 percent of your calories from fat per day.

• The Right Fit For You...or Not? While you are researching different diet plans, make sure it is something that you think would suit you and your lifestyle. If you are a very busy person who is not home a lot, look for a plan that has convenience as well as healthy choices. If you wind up choosing a plan that you don't stick to for whatever reason, you will wind up failing and you will then most likely go back to your old ways, but now feeling worse than when you started out.

• Calorie Level: Make sure that the plan you choose has you eating enough calories. You essentially want to cut out enough calories so that you can lose those 1-2 pounds a week. You have to weigh this all against you and your activity levels, as how many calories you need each day will vary from person to person depending on how active they are and their weight. You might want to work with a trained health professional to help you decide which is best for you.

How Diets Work

Losing weight is simple; lose more calories than you can eat.

We eat because it is a necessity. The food we consume will be processed by our body, breaking them down and only keeping what is needed while throwing out the rest. As we do our normal daily tasks our body uses calories and nutrients from our food as fuel for your body to complete all the tasks. However our body only needs a certain amount of calories to do this and this leads to all the unused calories being stored in our body as fat.

The problem with our body is there is no way to tell it to stop storing calories. All excess calories will be converted into fat no matter how much fat you have in your body already. Most of us would always eat more than we need to, taking in all those extra calories to lead us into being overweight.

"So in essence a diet is supposed to help you lose those extra calories"

A diet is an eating plan where you would control the amount of calories eaten. Eating less is not the only way to diet. Since the goal is to eat fewer calories, you can have constant food but it is low on calories. So foods like fruit or vegetables are low on calories if you compare same amount with other food like meat.

When you are dieting, you will be eating less than normal. So you would feel hungrier throughout the day and feel more unsatisfied when you finish your meal. It cannot be avoided since you are after all trying to lower your calorie intake. Do not be mistaken with skipping meals or starving yourself. Those will only worsen your diet conditions.

Beyond the Diet with Healthy Diet Recipes
What a good diet would include is help in suppressing the hunger, may it be psychologically or physically. Diet will always prepare you psychologically first before starting it. This is to ensure that you will be able to keep on the diet plan for the whole duration and reach your goal. Diet plans will also give you alternatives snacks that you can eat to suppress your cravings.

When you are on a diet, don't think that you will be having water and vegetables to last for the whole day. Diet actually promotes eating a balanced meal. You only want to have a lower calorie count but the rest of the nutrients shouldn't be ignored.

So when you are avoiding certain kind of foods, you would also be avoiding their nutrients. So the diet plan will show you alternative food you can take to replace the missing nutrients. Usually these foods are avoided and not forbidden completely. So you can still eat them in small portion once a while.

A good diet also contributes to your natural metabolism. Each person has his own rate of metabolism. A person with higher rate of metabolism will be able to burn more calories a day. A proper diet plan can help people with low metabolism to fully utilize them.

Like having a proper breakfast to jump start the metabolism, lunch to keep the energy going and eating less for dinner since you do not burn as much calories at night. This is to ensure that you have enough calories for the day.

Rule of Thumb

When you want to keep a diet plan, discipline is one of the most important factors. Weight loss through proper diet will take from months to years to achieve your proper weight. Diet that is extreme and promote speedy result can turn into a form of yo-yo dieting. Yo-yo dieting is a term where a person following a diet and manage to lose his weight but eventually will eat and gain more than he lose.

This happens because the diet he followed was too extreme; limiting his food intake and forbidding a lot of food category. So he cannot take all these diet thus giving in and eating more. Or it can be due to the lack of discipline after the targeted weight is achieved. This is usually the cause when you go for extreme hyper caloric diet.

So to avoid that, dieters are advised to go slow in their dieting where it will take months to see big result and where majority will quit halfway. It is not easy to change a habit you built up for years. So that is why you need a lot of discipline, willpower and determination to be able to stay on a diet.

Changing a habit is hard at first. You must stick to your diet plan daily for the first month. This will set the foundation. After 30 days it is said you have formed a new habit

No one has to diet alone. I truly encourage you to get a friend to help or even diet with you. By having someone beside you for encouragement, you can also slowly see the result in each other. It also helps to have someone to confide in when you think that the diet is not working out for you.

When you pick a diet to follow, you should consider a few diet plans that might be similar to the one that you are already doing. This is to diversify the diet. Following the same diet that you hate over and over again will have a negative effect on your willpower later on.

This might even cause you to abandon your diet. So by diversifying your diet, you will find a diet plan that you'll like and won't feel bored watching what you eat. You can cycle diet plan by weekly or monthly, making the diet eating plan fresh.

Just remember if you have broken one of your diet meals, this does not mean your whole day is ruined and you should not continue to follow your diet plan for the rest of the day. Just continue your day as if you never broken your diet in the first place. Over time this is what leads to long term weight loss/management

Industry Secrets

There are several things that the weight loss industry is not telling you – nor do they want you to know. Their business is booming thanks to all the fads, gadgets and pills out there that they are selling to people desperate to lose weight. Unfortunately, the only thing in most cases that is getting lighter is peoples' wallets. Many of these things do not work, and only a small percentage of people buying into one of them manage to lose the weight and keep it off.

Some of These Industry Secrets Include:

• Most weight loss product ads deceive the buyer. A majority of the weight loss products you hear about on the radio and see on infomercials don't even do what they claim to. Even so, consumers are lured into buying these products with promises like "Lose the weight and keep it off", "Eat whatever you want" and "no diet or exercise required". Basically, if it sounds too good to be true, it most likely is.

• Just because they say it's "scientifically proven" or "doctor-endorsed" doesn't mean it works. These claims are typical as well, but they never tell you anything about where the studies were made or by who so that you can check out the validity for yourself.

And what does it really mean anyway? Often these so-called health professionals have a financial interest in the product, and probably did not review the scientific evidence. If it was reviewed, they may not have even used acceptable review standards. Why would you want to risk your health on such a thing?

• Just because the government allows a product to be on the market does not mean it is safe for consumers or that it does what it claims. There is a huge misconception that the government would not allow a product on the market if it could potentially be harmful to you. People tend to think that the government has to pre-approve them first, but many times that is not the case.

• Products toted as 'natural' or 'herbal' are not guaranteed safe. People also assume that just because a product is made of natural ingredients means it must be safe as well. But until the FDA receives evidence that a product is harmful, the companies are free to put their products on the market.

Not everything you hear is true, and you shouldn't believe it. There are plenty of products that claim to do things that they just do not, and you should steer away from products making high and lofty claims.

Don't buy into the claims of fad diets, either. Anything that requires sudden and radical changes to your eating patterns is very difficult to sustain over time.

They will send you into a quick cycle of weight loss which is always followed by a rebound period where you gain the weight back and then some in certain instances once you're normal eating resumes.

Plus, the next time you try to take the weight off, it makes it all that much more difficult. There are no health benefits to these diets, and if any one of them worked, do you really think there would be the need for new ones?

You also can not count on the money back guarantee. You have about as good of a chance on getting your money back as having the product actually do what it claims to.

There is also no quick fix or magic pill that will help you to finally lose weight. If the product is making such claims, you can just about guarantee that they won't work.

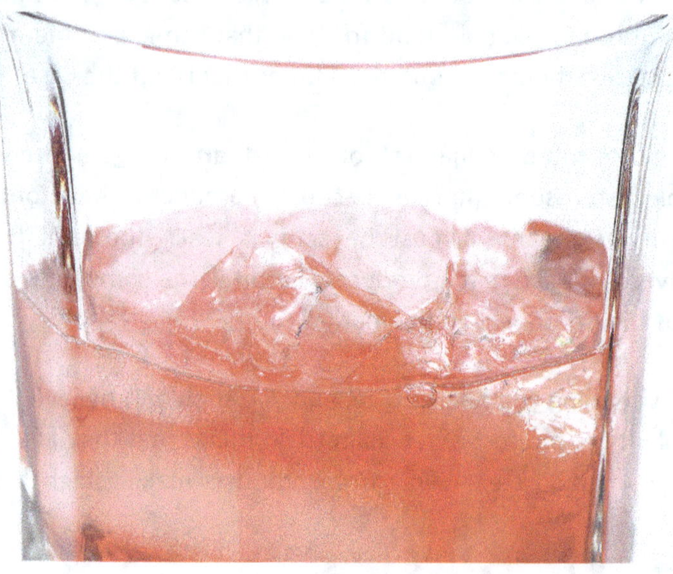

Chapter 2- Create an Action Plan to a Healthy Diet

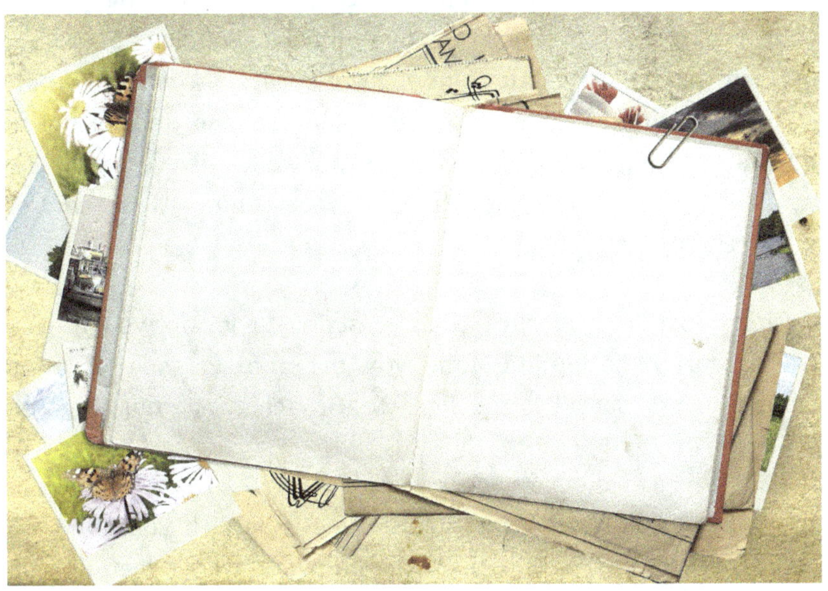

To make any diet a successful one, you need to be committed to it. Only with a right mind set can you reach success. To prepare yourself, you need to know what stage you are in before you can move on the next stage of your diet. It might not be obvious but it is there.

The First stage is pre-contemplation. You do not see yourself as being overweight. You do not feel like changing yourself. Only strong pressure will lead you to seek help. But then you would resist and just be demoralized as you see your own situation as hopeless.

Second is contemplation. This is where you acknowledge that you have an overweight problem and start to think of a solution. But you are not willing to perform that solution. You would just brood over it, knowing what actions to take to make a change but never ready to do so. You will procrastinate about performing the solution.

Third is preparation. You've finally decided to do something about your overweight problem. You move on from brooding about your problem to realizing your solution. You would also start to think about the future where you are slimmer and feeling much healthier. But at this stage you are not fully resolved yet. You would still have second thoughts about the solution as it requires you to change your lifestyle.

Fourth is action. You start to take action in losing weight. You would start choosing the food you eat and do some form of exercise every day. It is the first step in achieving your targeted goal.

You should always set goals when losing weight. If you don't set your goals, then it's very possible that your whole dieting plan might not go the way you imagine it.

"If you fail to plan, you plan to fail"

List the following:

• What is your current situation right now? List all your eating habits, food preferences, everything that could affect your weight loss. Working out, etc

• What is the reason you want to lose weight? This could be an upcoming event, summer, or even for a certain special someone. List the single BIGGEST reason you can think of.

• What are the benefits you get from your weight loss? List AS MANY as you can. It can be health, better energy, admired by partner, etc. This should be your main motivator.

• Your Goal. "I want to lose XX lbs of weight in XX days" - Write this in bold and make it really sink in. I would personally say that setting a goal of more than 10 lbs per 2 weeks is not realistic, especially if this is your first attempt at a goal like this. Be realistic. You must write "I want" not "I wish"

Write everything down and look at that paper every day. Put it in a place where you can see it. Once you see it every day, you will constantly be reminded of WHY you do this and what the benefits are.

BE PERSISTENT ONCE YOU TAKE ACTION BECAUSE IT'S NOT GOING TO BE EASY

STEPPING OUT OF YOUR COMFORT ZONE

If you see yourself making excuses rather than STARTING a diet that is effective, you should think about why you don't really want to lose weight. You must be able to step out of your comfort zone and as Nike's famous slogan goes JUST DO IT!

The final step would be maintenance. You need to keep the momentum going that you have in the action stage. If at any time you lose your commitment or support, then you would fall back to any of the previous stages.

So the final stage is the most important stage in your diet plan as you need to keep your commitment going for a long period of time. There are several methods you can use to keep being committed. First is to make a list about the reason why are you doing this in the first place. Look at the list daily to remind you of your goals. Do not have negative thoughts in your mind. Words like "never" or "depriving" should not be in your vocabulary. Rather than saying "never", you are just having desserts "occasionally and in moderation". And so the word "deprived" can be replaced with the word "choosing" as you choose to skip chocolate cakes.

Visualize in your mind your future slim self doing all the things that you always wanted to do. This visualization will strengthen your motivation to commit to this plan and be the desire to succeed. Do this visualization daily, every time you wake up and anytime of the day you feel your commitment is weakening.

Who to Approach When You Want to Lose Weight

Now that you've decided you want to lose weight, you should include some other people in your weight loss journey. These people can help you with many aspects, including choosing your diet plan, setting your goals and encouraging you along the way.

• A Therapist: Some people know they overeat, and how unhealthy it is for them as well, yet can't seem to stop their overeating no matter how hard they try. Many of these people eat for emotional reasons like loneliness or unhappiness and will try to hide their hurt and other feelings with food.

People that do this should seek the council of a therapist or other professionals trained in this specific matter so they can get the proper support. In some severe cases, it will take checking themselves into a specialized clinic designed for this purpose so that their nutrition and exercise can be closely monitored.

• A Dietician: A dietician will have a wide range of knowledge that can help you to understand your body and to help prepare a food plan that will fit your particular needs, because in most states and countries it is required to get a medical license before they can become a dietician.

Their goal is to help you eat healthier, and in turn you can lose weight. Because of this, dieticians are set apart from anyone who promotes a fad diet because they are not necessarily nutritionally sound for you. A dietician will also help you to figure out how many calories you need to consume in a day and to balance your intake of all the various food groups that you should be eating from.

• A Physical Trainer: The majority of people have never learned to exercise properly. A physical trainer will ensure that you do, and will push you to attain your goals, and can also help in the process of setting your goals. They will oversee your exercise routine in a gym, giving you both cardio and strength based exercises to follow.

The main goal of a personal trainer is to see to it that you get fit, and they also educate you on how to do that properly for yourself. Each person is different in their needs, and a personal trainer can adjust your training program to fit you just right. Over the course of the weight loss process, both the physical trainer and the dietician may give you advice in changing up your diet and your workout routine as you begin to gain more muscle tone to help support your new muscles.

• Friends and Family: When starting your weight loss journey, you may want to let friends and family know what you are doing so that they can be supportive of you. It always helps to have people you know and trust that stand by your side in any endeavor.

You can even have a friend or your spouse, keep you accountable to them and stop you from sneaking any extra snacks or sweets, or to motivate you to keep on your exercise regimen. You will likely be more successful in the end if you have someone alongside you (even over the phone if they are long distance) who will help encourage you when you are reaching your goals and to help push you when you start to struggle. Then, when you do reach your final goal (or even mini goals throughout) you can celebrate your achievements with the ones you love.

Persisting Through Failure

If you want to commit to losing weight, then you need to be able to persist through failure. Everyone who has accomplished something of note has struggled with failure at one or more points in their ascent. The difference is they didn't quit when it got tough, persisted through it and learned a lesson.

"When the going gets tough, the tough get going"

Those are the two keys in dealing with failure. You must persist and learn.

If you slip on your diet, or miss a day of exercise, don't fret about it. Don't let it derail you. Push it from your mind. Focus on all your positive days, not the one slip up.

Remember it is all about living a healthy lifestyle, the more good days add up and before you know it bad days become few and far between. But the trick is to keep going and push through the bad days. Treat it as a cheat day and move on. This is how you persist; failing for a day is OK, just don't let that day stretch into a week and then a month.

You have to accept failures as natural and develop a tough mental state to deal with them.

The second step is to learn from your mistakes. Quite often learning from your mistakes will be more efficient than learning from your successes. When you fail, treat it as a lesson learned. It is just like in business, when you fail at something, you learn the things that don't work. This is the same with weight loss. If you have slipped off your new diet every time you drink, then maybe you avoid drinking. If you realize that every Friday you miss out on exercise because of a late work meeting then reschedule your workout.

"I have not failed. I've just found 10,000 ways that won't work."

—Thomas A Edison

Failure is natural part of life, along with death and taxes. You can't avoid it, and even if you could you wouldn't want to. Your life's lessons are learned through your failures along with your successes. Don't fear failure, persist through and learn from it.

Buddy System

One of the best things you can do when you are trying to lose weight is to add some accountability to your routine. How do you do that?

The buddy system

Having a buddy to try and lose weight with is a great motivator. You will feel more accountable to reach your weight loss goals when you are actually sharing them with someone. They can also be helpful because the person is someone that can relate to you about struggling to lose weight. You can share your triumphs in joy, and your setbacks in support.

If you are working out regularly a buddy is invaluable. They can change a boring walk or jog into an exercise slash therapy session. A hike in the wilderness is always more fun with a friend along! If you are into weight lifting it is also nice to have a buddy. You guys can challenge each other while at the same time providing encouragement and practical help like spots on heavy lifts.

It is sad to say but in this day and age, you can probably find yourself a weight loss buddy in your group of friends. If you can't, don't panic you can always do it virtually online as well. You could find a friend on Facebook that is losing weight and work with them. Having Facebook chats and sharing progress pictures on Facebook.

There are also many web forums and sites dedicated to linking weight loss partners up virtually.

The bottom line is this - if you want to lose weight working with a friend can provide motivation, support as well as the always important accountability. Find your weight loss buddy now!

Why Maintaining a Daily Schedule is Critical

The next step in planning your weight loss goals is to set up a daily schedule for yourself. You need to decide when the best time for you to exercise is. For instance, if you are not a morning person, getting up two hours earlier than you are used to is probably not a good plan because you are likely to miss many mornings.

At the same time, if your job causes you to work late into the evenings frequently, scheduling your workouts for after work is not a wise idea either. You can also schedule out your meals, including the times you eat each day, and schedule out what your meals will be. The best thing to do is to schedule them out for a week at a time, and make a list and stick to it, so when you go shopping you will not be as tempted to impulse buy or stray off of your diet.

• Keeping Yourself in Check: If you have a specific schedule to follow, you are more likely to stick to your goals by writing everything down in a journal or other recording device like a smartphone. But, if you do miss a scheduled workout, or have an extra snack, you can keep note of it and vow to do better the next time.

• Knowing What You Are Doing Each Day: Having what time you are supposed to be doing your workouts or eating your meals written down can keep you in the know ahead of time, and in this way you can schedule things around your workout times, rather than scheduling over them and just missing workouts altogether. This can be easy to do, and if you start doing this, it will eventually snowball into increased times where you are missing your workouts, until you are thrown off track completely.

• Lose More Weight: By keeping yourself on a schedule, you will tend to lose more weight in the end because you will be likely to not miss any workouts (or very, very few in the long run). If you keep going back and forth and missing your workouts, or skipping a meal and confusing your body's metabolism, you will have a much harder time maintaining a steady rate of weight loss.

Chapter 3- Essential Benefits of Healthy Diet

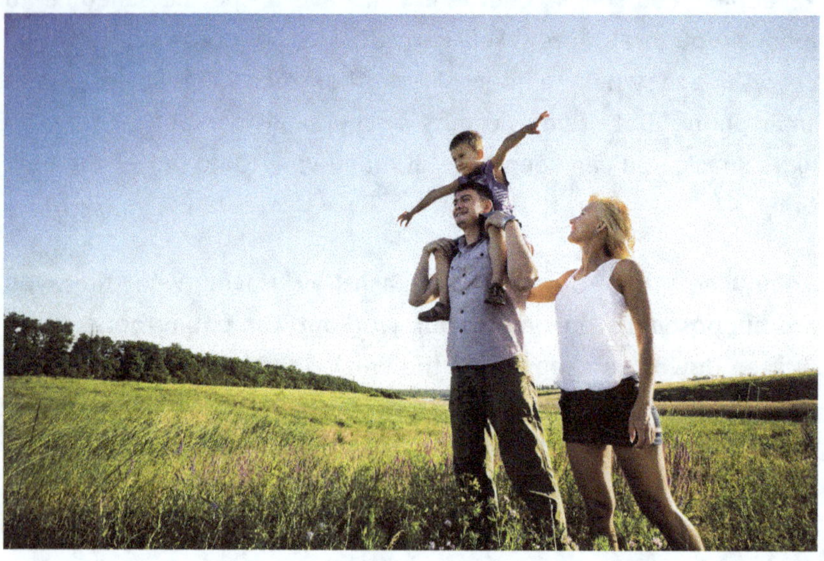

You would have heard lots of people saying that healthy nutrition is important for a healthy body but you need to know what the actual meaning of healthy nutrition is and why it is so important. Let's define nutrition.

"Nutrition is the process of giving your body all the important and necessary elements which can help it to grow in a proper and balanced way."

This is the simplest definition of nutrition which tells you that you need to eat proper food with good basic nutrients. Healthy nutrition can make your body strong and healthy also it can help it to grow and repair itself while an unhealthy nutrition plan can make your body weaker and can make you ill and you will not be able to fight against certain minor diseases.

Calories in - Calories Out

Everyone who wants to lose weight has probably tried multiple diets, supplements and/or plans. There are hundreds of weight loss methods available to buy. All of them making wild promises.

Here is the hard truth - there are no magical pills, diets or exercise gadgets that will make weight instantly disappear. It comes down to eating right, staying healthy and burning more calories than you take in.

That is where the saying "calories in - calories out" comes from. You want to make sure you burn more calories (out) than you consume (in).

Clearly, this is a simplistic view and a proper diet consists of taking more than calories into consideration. We will look at that in other chapters, but right now we want to talk about creating a calorie deficit.

In order to track this you need some basic information. First off you need to figure out how many calories you burn per day naturally. This comes down to factors such as age and weight.

Calculating the Number of Calories You Burn Daily

BMR calculation for men (kg)   BMR = 66.5 + (13.75 x weight in kg) + (5.003 x height in cm) − (6.755 x age in years)

BMR calculation for men (pounds)   BMR = 66 + (6.23 x weight in pounds) + (12.7 x height in inches) − (6.76 x age in years)

BMR calculation for women (kg)BMR = 655.1 + (9.563 x weight in kg) + (1.850 x height in cm) − (4.676 x age in years)

BMR calculation for women (pounds)   BMR = 655 + (4.35 x weight in pounds) + (4.7 x height in inches) – (4.7 x age in years)

This formula will give you the basic calories you burn daily, just by breathing, heart pumping and etc... These are how many calories you burn if you didn't move all day (basal metabolic rate).

Once you have that number, you need to start tracking the calories you burn and the calories you consume. This can be tricky because it is a lot of information to keep track of.

You just have to enter the foods and activity you had for the day. It will even allow you to input your basal metabolic rate.

It is ideal if you can keep a daily caloric deficit, but that isn't always possible. Sometimes we slip and sometimes we indulge. If you can get a weekly caloric deficit that will still have you losing weight.

This isn't about starving yourself, or exercising until you are dead. It is all about being aware what you put in your body, and what you exert. Weight loss can be a struggle, but if you can manage your calories in and calories out - you can overcome!

Clean Eating

We have talked about calories in calories out - the basic weight loss guideline. It is a basic tip because you still want to make sure you are getting those calories from good sources. Keeping your calories down by eating two corn-dogs a day probably isn't your best choice.

Eating clean is a term that doesn't have an official term but in general it means:

"Eating healthy whole foods while avoiding processed foods and refined sugars"

That is a general goal to strive for, it isn't always possible to eat completely "clean" but if you are getting the majority of your calories from clean sources then you are doing great. When you eat clean you avoid processed foods so automatically things like fast food and junk food are eliminated from your diet. If you do eat some processed food don't fret over it, the idea is to eat leanly as much as possible.

Here are some general clean eating tips:

• Learn to read labels! Read the nutritional information and ingredients of everything you buy.

• Choose while grains when possible. Whole wheat doesn't necessarily mean whole grain either! Look for bread, pasta and etc... Those are made with 100% whole grains

• Eat lots of fruits and vegetables. They are great whole sources of clean calories

• Prepare more of your own meals, don't eat out as much or buy microwaveable type meals. These meals even when "healthy", can be loaded with things like sodium.

• Choose lean meats when cooking. Eating meat is fine and the protein will help build muscle and make you feel full. Chicken and fish are great meat choices.

• Avoid processed meats like bologna or hot dogs.

• Replace junk food with unsalted or lightly salted whole nuts.

- Check out the internet for great clean recipes. Keep a list!

• Don't fret over falling off the wagon, even grat yourself a cheat day now and then.

• Eating clean while out can be tough but more restaurants are offering clean   menu items. A Salad can be a good choice, but if you are really hungry you might need to add some protein!

• Start as soon as possible!

Eating clean is a great way to make sure you not only lose weight but you are overall healthy. It isn't necessarily an easy transition and you don't have to try and turn on a switch and do it overnight. If you are committed to losing weight and being healthy, you should choose to clean up your diet.

Reducing Your Portions!

Anyone who is trying to lose weight needs to consider their portion control. Just talk to anyone who has actually lost weight (and sustained it). They will almost assuredly bring up portion control as one of the keys for their success.

What is Portion Control?

Portion control understands how much a serving size is and how many calories a serving contains.

One of the biggest problems overweight people face is realizing what constitutes a proper portion of food. When you eat a meal you need to realize what constitutes a serving size of your foods. While not scientific, the following list gives you an idea of some recommended portion sizes. If you struggle with weight loss, these portions might seem smaller than you thought:

• Vegetables or fruit is about the size of your fist.

• Pasta is about the size of one scoop of ice cream.

• Meat, fish, or poultry is the size of a deck of cards or the size of your palm (minus the fingers).

• Snacks such as pretzels and nuts are about the size of a cupped handful.

• Potato is the size of a computer mouse.

• Steamed rice is the size of a cupcake wrapper.

• Cheese is the size of a pair of dice or the size of your whole thumb (from the tip to the base).

I know personally that the cheese serving size surprised me when I first saw it. You can find portion information online. You can find much more specific portion control guides online as well. Some sites will break it down by food weight, so you may need to weight your food for exact portions. The above list though is good enough to give you a rough idea.

When you eat a meal, control your portions! Learning how much food you actually need is one of the biggest steps you will take on your weight loss journey.

Spreading out meals into smaller portions as opposed to eating enormous meals at any one time is a major factor in losing weight. It's been proven that rationing your meals not only reduces your caloric intake throughout the day but it also helps to steady your metabolism. If you're in the habit of eating 2-3 massive meals daily, consider eating 6-7 smaller meals which are spread out throughout your day.

One thing people enjoy doing is eating right from the packet as opposed to taking out what they need and putting the packet away. Such an example is eating out of a mega-sized packet of potato chips.

Not only do you have no idea how much you are consuming, but typically you're satisfying a craving by eating more than you really need until you are completely satisfied when instead you could pour a small portion into a bowl and add a piece of fruit to get the amount of food you actually need.

Super-sized packets are more commonplace now than before. More items are sold in bulk and more foods are served at restaurants with the option to supersize for a few extra cents. Increased portions are a factor in the rising statistics for obesity.

There is always a cause but people put enjoyment ahead of anything else which naturally leads to a health risk. This is why rationing meals are a handy way to take control of your bad habits.

It takes discipline to make adjustments and there's really no reason why people must feel they should eat until they're full. As always, tiny servings are fine and if still peckish, add a tiny bit more as opposed to loading your plate and trying to finish it all.

Rather than sit around feeling stuffed and undoing your belt buckle, leaving some room so that you can have another small meal a few hours later while still feeling good enough to mix in a little bit of exercise is a good balance which leads to improved results.

Doing this helps control the weight and slowly it begins to come down which is a marvelous feeling when you experience it, motivating you to work a little harder as you become confident in your ability to take control of your own body as opposed to allowing your cravings to take control for you.

Water Is Your Best Friend

It's been suggested by research that you require at least 8 glasses of water daily, but it can depend on your weight regarding how much you actually require. You would need to divide your weight by 2 so as an example, a man weighing 180lbs would need 60 ounces of water in a day.

So why do experts suggest that we drink lots of water and why is it considered so essential to a healthy life?

Well first off it helps to avoid dehydration and it keeps the kidneys functioning well by assisting in the elimination of waste products plus it helps to increase your metabolism which helps you to lose weight.

But aside from listening to what experts tell you, you should make it a priority to listen to your body first and foremost. When you are thirsty, then naturally you will drink water to replenish yourself.

Depending on the kind of work that you do, you should try to get into the habit of drinking water regularly or even better, keeping a water bottle handy, especially on really hot days since the heat causes you to sweat and your body loses water and thus you will need to replenish yourself.

This is why water is so important in our lives. Not only is it zero calories, it is the best source for quenching your thirst AND the healthiest.

You may consider adding water to all of your meals over time and doing away with fruit drinks and sodas ultimately as it will help reduce your caloric intake and you'll also feel much better without the added sugar that comes with the other drinks.

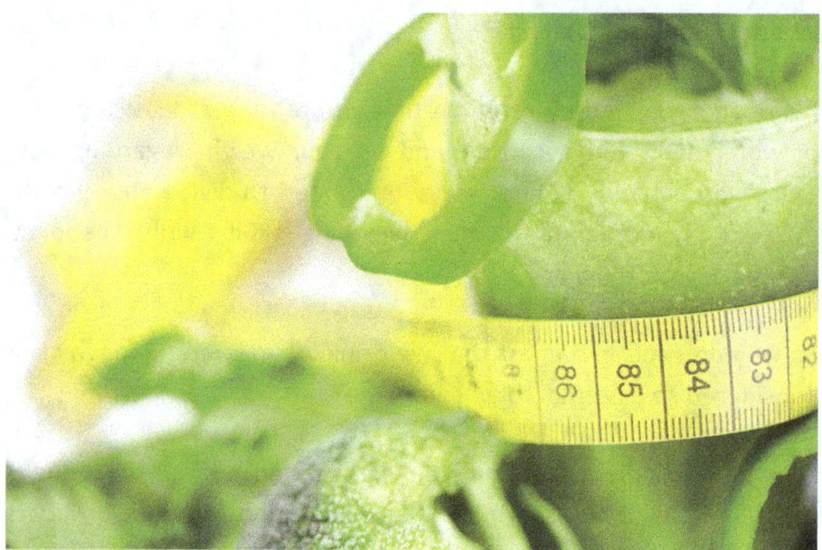

Chapter 4- Role of Exercise to a Healthy Lifestyle

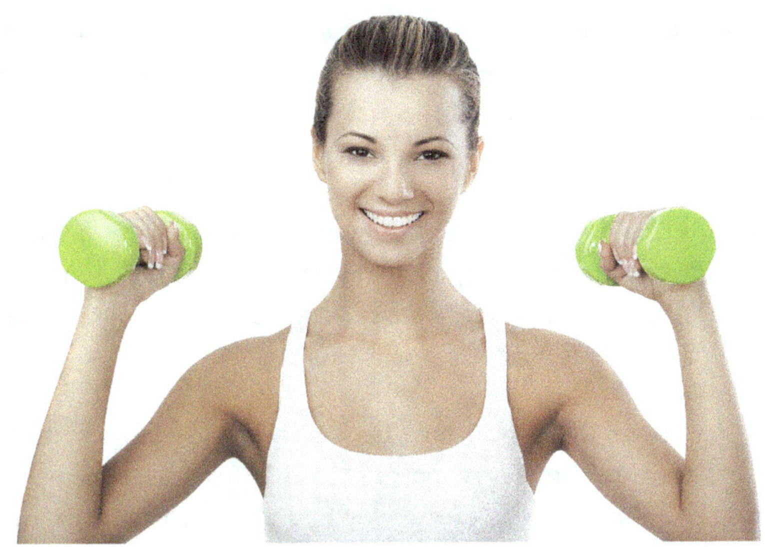

In this chapter, I will tell you about different types of exercises and their effects on different aspects of your life and health.

- Exercise to improve bone and muscle strength

- Flexibility increasing exercises

- Cardiovascular exercise

- Aerobics

Exercising

Exercising and dieting are two things that go hand in hand. If you just diet without exercising, you may not see any result at all because you are not losing calories fast enough in your diet. Also if you do manage to lose weight without dieting, you would look thin and frail as you lose your fat. So it is better to exercise to keep your body fit while you diet. There are also other reasons to exercise.

"A recent survey showed that seven out of ten adults do not exercise regularly and close to four out of ten are not physically active. If you do not exercise, then you will risk getting stroke, diabetes and heart disease. This has lead to death for about 300 000 people."

Before you start exercising, you should consult a physician. This is to know your current body condition and see if you would risk injuries if you perform tiring exercise activities. When you first start out exercising, do it slowly.

First start off with only 10 minutes which then is increase to 20 minutes then to 30 minutes and so on and so forth over the period of months. This will help avoid your body to feel very sore after each work out and decrease any injury risk.

You should at least do 30 minutes or more of moderate cardiovascular activities each day. You do not have to do all 30 minutes together; it can be even short bouts of intermittent activities.

Then twice a week, do exercise that would train your muscles. You can incorporate this physical exercise into your daily life. For example, take the stairs to the office instead of the elevator; go for a jog during your lunch time or park further away from your work place.

If you feel this is a too much of a chore, why not try to make your leisure time more active. Instead of sitting at home only, ask your family out for a bicycle ride, join a rock climbing club or just stroll the park every evening.

Pick out exercising activities that you would enjoy to do, find it satisfying and gives you a feeling of accomplishment. A successful run will motivate you more to be physically active. Make it easy for you to be active by picking exercise that is easier accessible so you will not be unmotivated every time you want to perform your exercise. Lastly, pick out exercise that is compatible with your body and current age.

The 3 Main Types Of Exercise

First of all, you need to know that there are three kinds of exercise plans which are available and all four of them have different advantages for your physical health.

Exercise To Improve Bone and Muscle Strength

These exercises are also called strength and resistance training. Most of the people take body building as strength and resistance increasing exercise but you need to know that body building is another category of exercise in which the primary goal of the person is to enhance muscle growth.

You can add some weight lifting and body building in your fat burning and weight control plan but you should do it to an extent where your body can bear it without any problem. If you over tried this exercise then, your whole body can be a mess.

I have seen people joining gyms and doing hard exercise just by watching other people doing it. This is not the way to go instead consult your trainer personally and ask him about appropriate exercises which can fit in your needs.

If your weight is under control and you need just light exercise to keep your healthy system going then, you do not need to lift heavy weights.

Flexibility Increasing Exercises

Second type of exercise plan can be to increase your flexibility and in more common terms you can say that if you used to have pain in your arms, legs, lower back, neck and other similar areas of your body then, you need to make your body more flexible. Flexibility will increase resistance and you will be able to cope with more difficult positions and postures easily.

You have to go through different postures in daily life for example if you work in an office then, you can be given an uncomfortable chair at times or you may be given some work in which you have to concentrate hard on computer screen and you cannot rest your back with chair. In these situations, if you do not have any flexibility in your body then, it will create problems but regular flexibility exercises which will not take more than 10-15 minutes of your time, will increase this flexibility and will make you feel better and active.

Cardiovascular Exercise

Cardio means heart and vascular means the vessels of blood and this whole phrase means that these exercises improve the functionality of your lungs and make the use of oxygen more effective and rectify any heart problems which you can have.

These exercises are little time consuming and should be properly learned from your doctor or trainer. Most of the times, people who already have got some heart problem perform these kinds of exercises to avoid any future problems.

Finding Exercises to Be Done At Home

A major change has been observed in the tendency of workout freaks, which is changing their exercise locale from gyms to home. Reason being, the soaring membership prices and binding contracts. As a result, they have started to opt for home fitness programs.

Finding exercises to be done at home is not a complex job, rather a much more convenient option. There are many great cardio exercises which can be done without much cost to the users.

The main money spent is in a good pair of walking, jogging or aerobic shoe, depending on the kind of activity desired. Besides, a jumping rope is also a great addition for skipping at home because it provides users added alternatives of aerobic workouts that can include rapid work interval training.

One can do it while watching TV or may be by playing music alongside. One should jump for a duration of thirty seconds to a minute as fast as possible and rest in between for sometime before starting again. You can always perform it during ad commercials and watch the rest of your show calming your body. Today, video and DVD market is flooded with exercise, aerobics and yoga CDs and DVDs which can be purchased for a favorable fitness exercise regime to start at home.

This gives more alternatives to people in case jogging or walking becomes mundane or if the weather does not allow you to go outside and run. Running and walking can actually become all the more interesting if done with a partner, provided no chit-chat and gossip hours begin and win over your fitness schedule. '

Varying the ground of the running or walking area can also add change to the daily workout process. Remember, it is very essential that you enjoy what you do to keep yourself fit if you actually want to feel the change in your health and body.

Besides, age does matter while selecting the kind of workout that you do. An adult person may be capable of losing weight using particular equipments and build muscles as well, but an elderly may not just get the same results from the same regimen. It is simply because of the quality of performance and not the utilization the expensive and similar machines. Thu, it's advisable that you always choose a kind of fitness regimen that goes well with your body, age and needs keeping the various health constraints that age brings along.

Exercises that you can perform at home

Leaving you with no excuses of not finding the right type of exercises that you can do at home, here is a list of the appropriate home fitness based program exercises for you-

• These exercises can be performed by using easy drills at home and employing minimal equipments which you can get from around your house.

• For upper body you can do chair dips, lateral raises, push-ups, chin ups and bent over row. For core exercises you can do dead lift, sit ups and Side Bridge.

• For lower body you can opt for step ups, wall squat, bucket squats and lunges.

Prior to starting these exercises you must warm up yourself for minimum of five minutes by jogging or brisk walk around the block or by skipping on the spot. You must perform multiple sets of the exercises mentioned above depending upon your endurance level and requirement. Also, taking intervals in between is equally essential. You can combine two exercises that use diverse muscle groups alternating between two things that provide each muscle group some rest while you perform another.

To get the best results, perform these workouts at least three times a week, with no less than a day between exercises for sufficient recovery. You must always strive to increase the intensity or load and to increase your fitness growth. Once your fitness improves, you can undergo this routine without bothering much and start with a more superior program. Use your creativity and find more things to use for working out at home.

Using buckets, filled with the amount of water you want can be employed for squats and step-ups.

Filling up milk bottles with 2 liter water makes it equivalent to a 2 kg weight to be used for overhead triceps extension, bicep curls and bent over rows.

Shopping bags and backpack filled with items can be used for lunges, step-ups and squats. Utilizing bricks by breaking them in half in case of lower weight is appropriate for pushups, bench press, lateral raises and front raise.

Then comes the age old forms of exercises that come under the practice of yoga asana a lot of people not just perform these exercises for the sole aim of relieving mental stress but to get and stay fit as well. If you look at the fitness regimens of every famous celebrity today including the big names like Jennifer Aniston, Drew Barrymore, it is yoga that has worked wonders on their body to get the envious figure every girl wants.

Not only women, even men have also started incorporating this form of fitness to build up muscles using their own body weight. This is the most natural way of dealing with your body and respecting it as well.

Chapter 5- Tips on How To Live a Healthy Lifestyle

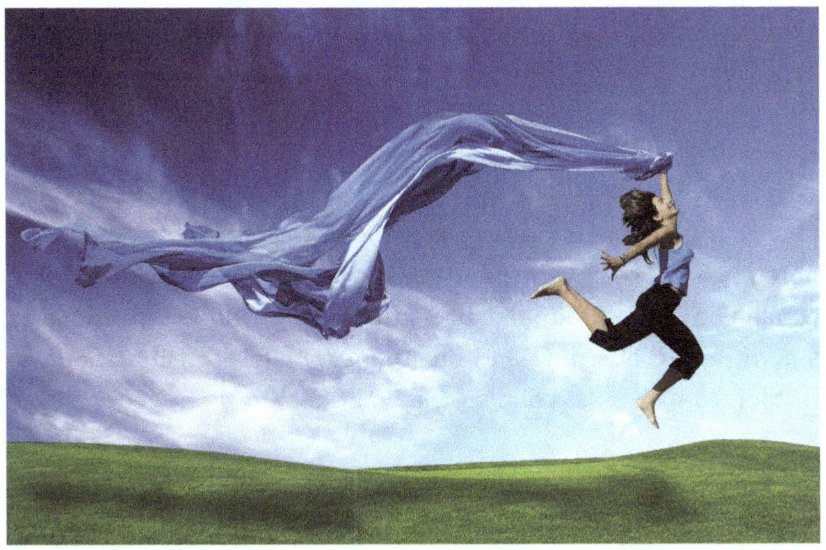

Once you have reached your target weight, you'll want to know how to maintain it so you don't put all that hard work to waste! Educating yourself ahead of time will help you when you are at the point where you have attained your weight loss goal. You wouldn't want to ruin the celebration you will want to have, and you of course want to continue on with your newfound healthy lifestyle.

• Don't skip any meals! Remember, your body's metabolism will take this as a signal that your body is starving and will begin to store fat for reserves. Make sure you keep up with eating your meals, scheduled out as you have been. Besides, if you skip a meal at one point in the day, it could mean you overeat later on when you are just so hungry.

• Keep eating a variety of foods. This will help you to keep getting all the nutrients and vitamins your body needs to stay working properly. It will keep you feeling healthy, energized and protect your body by keeping it healthy. You can include choices from whole grains, fruits, vegetables and lean proteins.

• Keep up the exercising! Don't get lazy and slack off on your exercise routine now. You have gained the knowledge of what kind of a workout is right for you, and probably how to change it up every once in a while as well if you had instruction from a personal trainer.

Changing up your routine is a great idea to keep you from getting bored, and to keep your body guessing. As long as you are always combining your cardio and strength training, you will continue to stay fit and feel strong and healthy, all while protecting yourself further from illnesses coupled with your healthy diet.

• Adjust your daily caloric intake. Many people wonder if they should increase their daily caloric intake right away. It is probably advisable to do so, but do so gradually. Try starting with just 250 calories more a day.

After a week, weigh yourself. You'll probably still have lost some more weight. If this is the case, add another 250 calories, then weight yourself a week after that. Repeat these steps until you see that your weight has remained the same when you weigh yourself for the week. If you gained a bit, take away some calories, 100 at a time, until your weight evens out and remains the same from week to week.

• Keep drinking that water! Don't forget to have at least eight glasses of water a day to keep your body working well. Water aides in digestion, increases your energy and helps rid your body of toxins naturally. Plus, you will stay hydrated and healthy.

• Keep eating frequently. Eating five to six small meals a day as you have probably already learned to do is a good thing to continue doing, as this keeps your metabolism up, and keeps you feeling satisfied. It is important to continue this as well because you don't want to fall into the trap of increasing your portion sizes again if this was a problem before. You will throw yourself all the way back to square one eventually. In the very least, you will gain a bunch of the weight back you worked so hard to shed.

• Don't let the junk food back in. Now that you've developed your healthy habits, why ruin it by going back to your old ways and eating junk food? You have discovered plenty of delicious tastes to satisfy all your cravings with healthy foods. Keep your intake of fruits and vegetables up to several servings a day, preferably 6-8.

• Take your daily vitamins. Remember to keep taking your daily vitamins as well. Doing this will help assure that you acquire all the vitamins you need each day and it will help you to maintain your healthy weight as well.

The Secrets of Staying Healthy

Everybody wants to live long and healthy lives; nobody wants to count on getting any severe diseases. Although we can't predict or prevent every situation, there are ways to help protect ourselves that can make our lives more full and healthy overall.

• Prevention and early detection is the first thing you should consider. Most people dread going for a yearly physical, or even the dentist cleaning every six months, but having good doctors and keeping these appointments in your life will help you to stay healthy because you doctor can detect things that you can't on your own.

Knowing your family history is also important because if there is any history of heart disease or cancers in your family your doctor can keep any eye out for symptoms and do testing on you regularly.

• Love the people you are with. Make sure and spend time with the ones who surround you daily such as your spouse, children, other family members, friends and coworkers. Enjoy the time you spend with other people, plus maintain healthy friendships. These relationships are needed to make you feel fulfilled in life.

• Get eight hours of sleep. Although many people find this one difficult to do because of how busy we can get in our lives, it really is very important to leading a happy and healthy life.

• Find something you are good at. All of us have times where we need to be doing something we really enjoy, and most of these are things that we excel at. This is usually something that makes us feel good inside as well, and can even be soothing and stress relieving.

• Manage your stress – don't ignore it! Everyone has stressors of some kind, and it is important that we handle our stress so that it does not get out of hand and consume us.

When you are riddled with worry and stress it can literally make you sick in many different ways. Daily walks can help clear your head, and make sure that you are not over-filling your agenda for each day or letting other's schedules dictate your day.

• Find balance in your life. Don't try to take on too many projects at work or let work consume you. Find a balance so you are still able to enjoy all the other things around you like your hobbies and your friends and family.

Although financial times can be tough, it is still so very important to find time to spend at least with your family, the ones you are working so hard to keep safe and provided for.

The Advantages of Staying Healthy

The benefits of staying healthy are boundless. It doesn't just mean that you are happy with the way you look and can fit into that new outfit. Being healthy has to do with your whole physical, mental and social well-being.

• Your Physical Health: Keeping yourself physically healthy can help you all around. Not only can it help you to take part in daily activities such as being able to walk, move and bend, but it allows you to be physically able to take care of your loved ones around you who depend on you.

It can be financially beneficial if you avoid diseases that were preventable and that would be very costly.

• Your Mental Health: If you do not have a good mental health, your physical health will also be affected. Many people don't realize just how important their mental health is to their overall well-being. If you allow yourself to be over-stressed or for that stress to rule your life, it can make you sick.

Stress can raise your blood pressure which increases your risk of a heart attack or stroke. You need to deal with your stress in positive ways like through exercise, meditation or therapy. Don't deal with stress by things that can damage your overall health like smoking, drinking or eating unhealthy foods.

• Disease Prevention: Making sure you are eating a healthy diet is vital to your overall health and staying healthy. The foods you choose to eat can have a direct impact on your health.

Phytochemicals are important for your health and could prevent things like heart disease, specific types of cancer, diabetes and high blood pressure. They are found only found in certain foods like berries, spinach, olives and kale. Eat a low-fat diet full of lots of fruits and vegetables plus whole grains to help protect your cardiovascular health.

• Long Life: Striving to live a healthy lifestyle can be a big factor of you being able to live a long and healthy life. Although you can't prevent all health problems and some of them are out of your control, a lot of the most significant ones you can help to avoid by living healthy.

With the leading causes of death being chronic diseases such as diabetes, heart disease, stroke and cancer, having lifestyle choices that include controlling the foods you eat, keeping your weight at a healthy level, how much you exercise and how you deal with the stressors in your life can have a huge impact on keeping these diseases at bay.

Living a healthy lifestyle can also improve your mood and give you greater self-esteem and mental focus. You will be stronger, have a higher stamina and you will be able to get a better night's sleep.

Other benefits of a healthy lifestyle include improved digestion and a lower blood pressure. Keeping yourself healthy can also help ease or eliminate back problems and back pain plus improve your posture, enhance coordination and balance, and lower your resting heart rate.

Chapter 6- Healthy Meal Plans – Healthy Diet

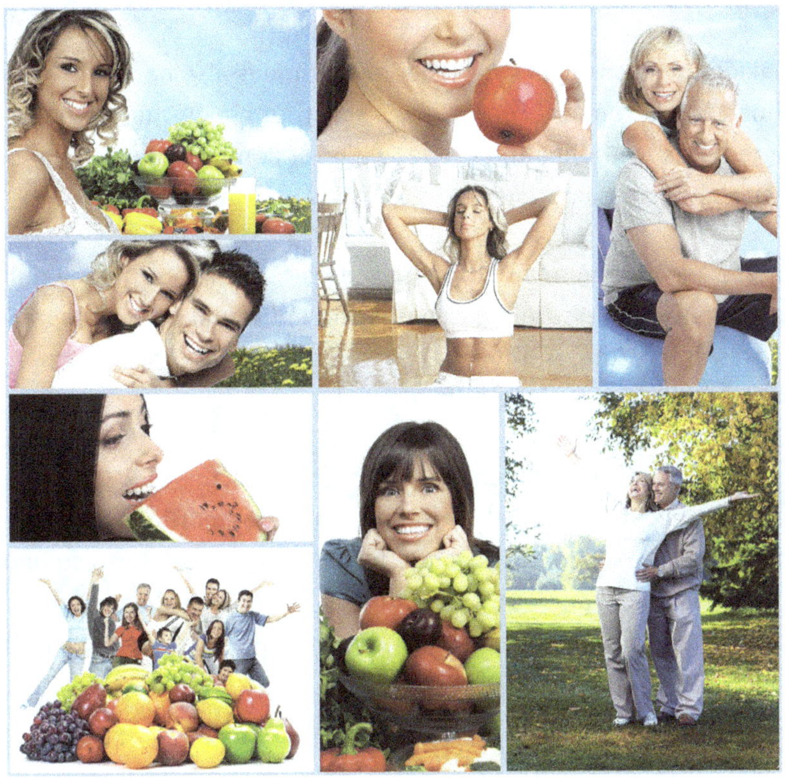

Ideally small amount of food intake is best but only if these amounts consists of nutritionally balanced and healthy elements.

Exploring the various nutritional basics of each category within the food groups helps the individual to make informed choices regarding the food consumed. Upon gaining this understanding the next step would be to make the changes needed but doing so gradually would better reap positive results as opposed to drastically making the change which the body may accept for a short period of time and then reject in the long run.

Beyond the Diet with Healthy Diet Recipes

Finding the foods in simpler and more variety and freshness though still maintaining some of the favorite ingredients helps the body accept the new food intake with less of a shock to the system both body and mind.

Making these changes over a period of time is also necessary if the effort is to remain continuous. Substituting certain unhealthy ingredients with healthier one while still maintain the general recipe is also recommended.

Totally avoiding unhealthy foods is of course ideal but really quite an unrealistic pressure as it causes the individual to feel deprived and stressed, therefore a better alternative would be to wean themselves slowly off the item instead.

Learning to eat in smaller portions also helps the individual start the journey towards healthy eating. For some cutting out certain foods may be such a difficult effort that the next best solution would be to try and cut down the portions. Also developing the habit of avoiding heavier meals towards the end of a day is also wise.

Black Bean Recipe

As more and more people become aware of this particular food called the black bean the interest in it has also become heightened. Originating from Mexico and very much a part of the South American diet, these black beans have been proven to be quite a nutritionally pack food group indeed. Today it is popularly found in most restaurants and homes in various forms such as salads, staples and other delicious dishes.

Black Beans

The black beans consists of high protein and fiber contents and is considered very nourishing as both these essential elements are present within one food item. Fiber and proteins are considered very important to the wholesome function of a healthy body. Besides this it also has flavonoid anti oxidants content which assist the body avoid oxygen related damage. Black beans also consists of omega 3 fatty acids and has a high nutritional value.

Black beans are also very easy to incorporate into most meals as it has a basic flavor of rich smokiness, which gives added character to any dish. The velvet texture, shape and color hold well during cooking and makes for a very interesting looking ingredient indeed.

Black Bean Salad Ingredients

The Salad - (I try to keep the cuts not too much bigger than the beans & corn - for appearance & to get a little of everything in a spoonful)

2 lbs. black beans (I have a pressure cooker, but go ahead, use 2 15 oz. cans, well-rinsed.)

2 lbs. cooked sweet corn, cut from the cob (OK, you can use 2 - 15 oz. cans of whole kernel corn or 2 lbs. of frozen corn, drained)

8 green onions, diced

2 cloves garlic, large, minced

2-3 jalapeno peppers, cleaned, diced (more if you like)

Beyond the Diet with Healthy Diet Recipes
1 green Bell pepper, cleaned, diced (I also sometimes add a small sweet red pepper, for both sweetness & color)

1 ripe avocado, large, pitted, peeled and diced 1 jar (4 oz) pimentos, drained

3 tomatoes, seeded & diced 1C fresh cilantro, chopped

Sea salt & fresh cracked black pepper to taste The Dressing

3 T fresh lime juice

2 T fresh orange juice 2-1/2 tsp lime zest 1/2 tsp ground cumin

Sea salt & fresh cracked black pepper to taste Directions

Combine all the salad ingredients in a large bowl. Season with the salt

& pepper. Whisk the dressing vigorously to incorporate. Add the dressing to the salad and gently toss to combine everything. Chill until ready to serve. Lightly toss again prior to serving.

Prepare this salad at least 4 hours prior to serving to let everything - except the avocado - marry joyfully in the bowl.

You do want to let the avocado bathe in the lime juice of the dressing - better presentation that way, and you can store the avocado pieces in a small container. Then, pour the dressing off the avocado and mix the salad with the dressing, then dress the top of the salad with the avocado pieces at service.

Very pretty dish & the absence of any oil seem to make all the veggies sparkle in a light citrus glow. You want this salad well chilled, but if you don't bathe the avocados in the dressing first, they will end up looking like grey lumps of pork as the air hits them.

Oat Recipe

Eating oats to enhance good health is not something new but has been practice through time. Oats is a very simple ingredient with far reaching positive effects and benefits.

Oats within a diet plan provides a wide range of important health benefits which cannot be duplicated by any other food item singularly. Being a significant dietary fiber source, oats consists of soluble and half soluble fibers which help to keep blood cholesterol levels effectively under control.

Some of the areas where oats has been known to be beneficial are in improving heart conditions, regulating blood sugar levels, functioning as anti cancer fighters, keeping blood pressure under control, maintaining regular and healthy bowel functions, helping in weight control, boosting athletic performances, and in general health and longevity. Oats

Oats is also a food item that is rather hardy and can be grown in poor soil conditions which is of course another plus in terms of its availability. The various processes that the oat has to be subjected to before it reaches the dining table does not cause its nutritional value to decrease rather it is able to maintain its concentrated high fiber and nutrient base.

Oats can be a great day starter in the form of a piping bowl of oatmeal which can be more flavorful with the addition of fresh fruits, nuts or the dried fruits variety. It can also be used to make oat meal cookies which are usually a huge hit with kids and adults alike. Breads and muffins can also have the addition of healthy oats to it as with poultry stuffing too.

Golden Honey Oat Bread Recipe

Ingredients

1   1/4 cups and 2 tablespoons water, room temperature (70 to 90°F.)

1/2 cup rolled oats or barley flakes 1/4 cup flax seed cracked

2   cups unbleached flour 3/4 cup whole wheat flour

2 tablespoons vital wheat gluten 1 tablespoon powdered milk

2 tablespoons honey

1 1/8 teaspoon instant yeast 2 1/2 tablespoons canola oil 2 teaspoons salt

Directions

Equipment: A 9 by 5 inch/ 7 cup bread pan, coated lightly with cooking spray. A baking stone set toward the bottom rung and a cast- iron pan on the floor of the oven.

Step 1: Make the dough (Bread Machine)

In the bread machine container, combine water, oats, and cracked flax and mix to moisten. Then let sit covered for a minimum of 15 minutes.

In a medium bowl, whisk together the flours, gluten, powdered milk, and yeast.

Add the honey, and oil to the oat mixture and then the flour mixture. Mix 3 minutes and allow to rest for 20. If your bread machine always restarts with a 3 minute mix allow it to do so while adding the salt and then go into the kneading cycle for 4 minutes. If it starts with the kneading cycle also run it for 4 minutes, adding the salt at the beginning of the kneading cycle.

Step 2: Let the dough rise

Using an oiled spatula or dough scraper, scrape the dough into a 2 quart container with cover or bowl, greased lightly with cooking spray or oil. Push down the dough and lightly spray or oil the top of the dough. It will be 4 cups /943 grams/33 ounces.). Cover the container with a lid or plastic wrap. With a piece of tape, mark where double the height would be.

Allow the dough to rise (ideally at 80 to 82°F/28°C) until doubled, about 1 hour, 15 min. For extra strength and elasticity, you can stretch it after the first 30 minutes. To achieve a moist and warm temperature I put a small container of very hot water—about 1 cup--under a plastic box to create a proofer and change the water every 20 to 30 minutes. (You can retard the dough overnight after the first rise by gently deflating it and refrigerating it but it seems to rise best when baked the same day. If you refrigerate it overnight, remove it to room temperature. For about an hour before shaping.

Step 3: Shape the dough and let it rise

Turn the dough onto a lightly floured counter and press it down to flatten it slightly. It will still be sticky but use only as much flour as absolutely necessary. Shape it into a log and allow it to relax covered for 20 minutes. (This is essential for evenly shaped dough.)

Shape the dough into a loaf set it into the prepared baking pan. It will be about 3/4 inches from the top of the pan.

Cover the shaped dough with the plastic box or oiled plastic wrap and allow it to rise until almost doubled and when pressed gently with a finger the depression very slowly fills in. The highest point will be about 1 1/2 inches higher than the sides of the pan. Using the plastic box and hot water it takes 1 hour 15 minutes to 1 1/2 hours. At a cooler temperature it will take longer. Meantime preheat the oven for a minimum of 40 minutes.

Step 4: Slash and bake the bread

If you like the look of a bread with a slash down the middle, with a sharp knife or straight edged razor blade, make a 1/2 inch deep slash down the top of the dough. You can also leave it unlashed. Mist the dough with water, quickly but gently set the baking sheet on the hot stone or hot baking sheet and toss 1/2 cup of ice cubes into the pan beneath.

Immediately shut the door, lower the temperature to 375ºF/190ºC, and bake 20 minutes. Turn the dough around, tent, and continue baking 15 to 20 minutes or until the bread is golden brown and a skewer inserted in the middle comes out clean. (An instant read thermometer inserted into the center will read about 205°F.)

Step 5: Cool the bread

Unmold the bread onto a wire rack and allow it to cool, top-side-up until barely warm.

Avocado Recipe

More and more today the world is looking to avocados as the next wholesome nutritious food replacement. Originating in Mexico and Central America it can now be found in many other countries like Indonesia, Philippines, Thailand, India, china, Japan, Peru and the list goes on.

Avocado

Ranging from being able to cure certain cancer diseases to the ideal food energy source for body builders, this remarkable fruit is fast gaining the popularity it so aptly deserves.

A little known fact about the avocado is that, when the avocado fruit is mixed into salads, it aids in the absorption of all the other nutrients the salad may have in a more efficient way.

When a comparison is made with other fruits the avocado wins all the time, as the fruit that is better able to allow the nutrients to be absorbed and also for its high content of many different nutrients.

The avocado is also considered a "meaty" fruit as the creamy like texture is rich and quite adequately makes for a good meal or an accompanying ingredient that enhances and enriches any dish.

For those wanting to avoid certain foods for health or religious reasons the avocado is known to be a good substitute as it contains adequate amounts of meat proteins, fat oils, vitamins and minerals.

Avocado Dip Ingredients

4 avocados

1 red onion

1/2 bunch of cilantro 1 ear of sweet corn

1 pint of sweet grape tomatoes Juice of 1/2 lime

2 fresh jalapeno peppers Directions

Remove avocado and dice in a bowl. Shuck corn and remove kernels from cob and add to avocado. Dice red onion, cilantro and jalapeno. Slice tomatoes in half. Add to mixture, season with salt and pepper. Cover with plastic wrap and store in fridge. Be sure to press plastic wrap to the surface of the dip to prevent browning. I also add the avocado seed to the bowl to help prevent browning.

Salmon Recipe

Consuming salmon in moderation has many health benefits, some yet to be fully explored but none the less accepted as one of the best and purest form of providing the fatty acid richness humans need. It is known to aid in the optimum health conditions that allows people to live longer and healthier lives.

The proteins found in salmon can easily be digested and absorbed into the body's system without causing any adverse effects that some other proteins have been known to cause.

The proteins which are found in the salmon are referred to as amino acids and are vital to the human health as these good fats or Omega 3 fatty acids provide the necessary balance for the body.

Salmon also has vitamin A, B and D, minerals, iron, phosphorus and selenium within the content makeup.

Salmon

For those having heart problems, or recovering from a heart attack, the consumption of salmon is encouraged primarily because it aids in the lowering of bad cholesterol and replacing it with good cholesterol. Salmon also helps to repair heart damage and strengthen the heart muscles. Salmon also works as a natural antidepressant and help the brain work better while improving the memory capabilities of an individual.

There is even some evidence of being able to positively affect the aging process. Salmon also helps to lower the blood sugar level which is especially beneficial to those suffering from diabetes. It also contributes to a more optimum metabolic rate. Healthy hair which is bright and shiny, good skin quality and bright eyes are all the positive benefits of consuming salmon.

Baked Salmon Ingredients

Fresh salmon filets (allow about 1 per person)

1/3 cup orange juice 2 lemons

Salt Pepper

Garlic powder Italian seasoning

Fresh cilantro for garnishing Directions

Preheat oven to 375 degrees

Wash & place salmon filets skin side down into deep rectangular baking dish

Mix 1/3 cup orange juice with the juice of one of the lemons; pour mixture over salmon filets in baking dish

Season each salmon filet with salt, pepper, garlic powder, and Italian seasoning to taste

Cut the second lemon in half, cut one half of lemon into slices and place slices on top of salmon filets

(The second half of this lemon will be sliced and placed on salmon after it's done)

Bake salmon filets for 15-25 minutes depending on the thickness after baking, place filets on serving dish and place slices from the second half of the lemon on top

Garnish filets with cilantro

Eating Right

There are a lot of good and delicious foods that are not only good for the body but it also have the added advantage of not causing the body to retain unwanted pounds through its consumption. There are also ways preparing foods that are less likely to cause weight retention and this too should be explored if the individual is unwilling to give up eating a certain food or ingredient.

Simple measures can be taken without causing too much of a shock to the body system in the initial stages. These adjustments can then be increased as and when the body is ready and able to accept more deprivation.

Drinking a lot of water and cutting out as much sweetened food items as possible is one of the first and simplest steps to take in the quest to keep the pounds off. Keeping a food diary may also help the individual to be more aware of the foods consumed, thus creating the opportunity for the individual to make the healthier choice whenever possible.

Enlisting the help of professional, such as doctors, health experts, dietitians, nutritionist can also help the individual better understand and accepts the negatives and positives of the current foods being consumed and then tailor make an appropriate diet plan with healthy food contents to encourage satisfaction without the added pounds.

Chapter 7- Healthy Diet Recipes

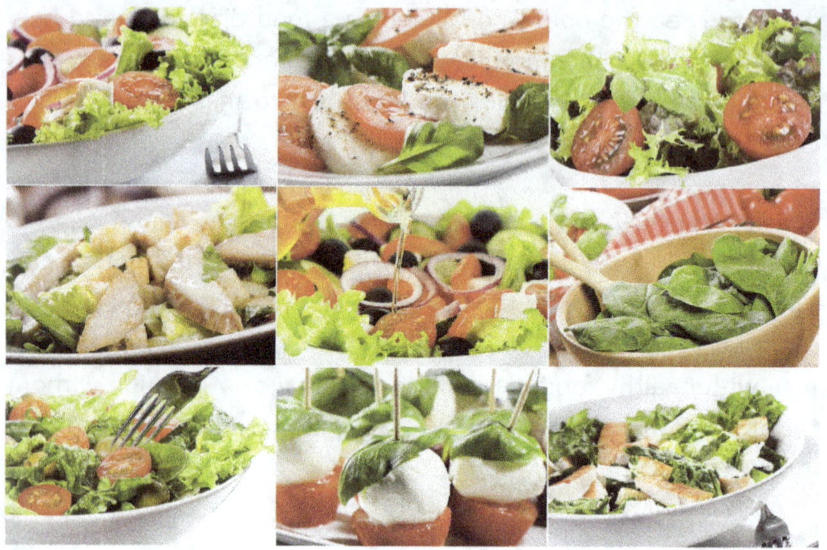

BOILED FISH

Boiling extracts flavor and, to some extent, nutriment from the food to which this cookery method is applied. Therefore, unless the fish to be cooked is one that has a very strong flavor and that will be improved by the loss of flavor, it should not be boiled. Much care should be exercised in boiling fish, because the meat is usually so tender that it is likely to boil to pieces or to fall apart.

When a fish is to be boiled, clean it and, if desired, remove the head. Pour sufficient boiling water to cover the fish well into the vessel in which it is to be cooked, and add salt in the proportion of 1 teaspoonful to each quart of water.

Tie the fish in a strip of cheesecloth or gauze if necessary, and lower it into the vessel of slowly boiling water. Allow the fish to boil until it may be easily pierced with a fork; then take it out of the water and remove the cloth, provided one is used. Serve with a well-seasoned sauce, such as lemon cream, horseradish, etc.

BOILED SALMON -1

This fish is seldom sent to the table whole, being too large for any ordinary sized family; the middle cut is considered the choicest to boil. To carve it, first run the knife down and along the upper side of the fish from 1 to 2, then again on the lower side from 3 to 4.

Serve the thick part, cutting it lengthwise in slices in the direction of the line from 1 to 2, and the thin part breadth wise, or in the direction from 5 to 6. A slice of the thick with one of the thin, where lies the fat, should be served to each guest. Care should be taken when carving not to break the flakes of the fish, as that impairs its appearance. The flesh of the salmon is rich and delicious in flavor. Salmon is in season from the first of February to the end of August.

BOILED SALMON -2

The middle slice of salmon is the best. Sew up neatly in a mosquito-net bag, and boil a quarter of an hour to the pound in hot salted water. When done, unwrap with care, and lay upon a hot dish, taking care not to break it. Have ready a large cupful of drawn butter, very rich, in which has been stirred a tablespoonful of minced parsley and the juice of a lemon. Pour half upon the salmon and serve the rest in a boat. Garnish with parsley and sliced eggs.

BOILED SALMON -3

When smoked salmon can be secured, it makes a splendid fish for boiling. If it is cooked until tender and then served with a well-seasoned sauce, it will find favor with most persons. Freshen smoked salmon in warm water as much as seems necessary, remembering that the cooking to which it will be subjected will remove a large amount of the superfluous salt. Cover the salmon with hot water, and simmer slowly until it becomes tender. Remove from the water, pour a little melted butter over it, and serve with any desired sauce.

BOILED SALT SALMON.

Let salmon soak overnight, and boil it slowly for two hours; eat it with drawn butter. To pickle salmon after it has been boiled, heat vinegar scalding hot, with whole peppers and cloves; cut the fish in small square pieces; put it in a jar, and pour the vinegar over. Shad may be done in the same way.

BOILED COD.

A fish that lends itself well to boiling is fresh cod. In fact, codfish prepared according to this method and served with a sauce makes a very appetizing dish.

Scale, clean, and skin a fresh cod and wrap it in a single layer of gauze or cheesecloth. Place it in a kettle or a pan of freshly boiling water to which has been added 1 teaspoonful of salt to each quart of water. Boil until the fish may be easily pierced with a fork, take from the water, and remove the gauze or cheesecloth carefully so as to keep the fish intact. Serve with sauce and slices of lemon.

BOILED SALT COD

Put your fish to soak overnight; change the water in the morning, and let it stay till you put it on, which should be two hours before dinner; keep it at scalding heat all the time, but do not let it boil, or it will get hard; eat it with egg sauce or drawn butter. If you have any

Cod fish left from dinner, mix it with mashed potatoes, and enough flour to stick them together; season with pepper; make it into little cakes, and fry them in ham drippings.

BOILED COD WITH LOBSTER SAUCE.

Boil the fish, as directed [see boiled fish], and, when done, carefully remove the skin from one side; then turn the fish over on to the dish on which it is to be served, skin side up. Remove the skin from this side. Wipe the dish with a damp cloth. Pour a few spoonfuls of the sauce over the fish, and the remainder around it; garnish with parsley, and serve. This is a handsome dish.

BOILED HADDOCK WITH LOBSTER SAUCE.

The same as cod. In fact, all kinds of fish can be served in the same manner; but the lighter are the better, as the sauce is so rich that it is not really the thing for salmon and blue fish. Many of the best cooks and caterers, however, use the lobster sauce with salmon, but salmon has too rich and delicate a flavor to be mixed with the lobster.

BROILED FISH -1

The best way in which to cook small fish, thin strips of fish, or even good-sized fish that are comparatively thin when they are split open is to broil them. Since in this method of cooking the flavor is entirely retained, it is especially desirable for any fish of delicate flavor.

To broil fish, sear them quickly over a very hot fire and then cook them more slowly until they are done, turning frequently to prevent burning. As most fish, and particularly the small ones used for broiling, contain almost no fat, it is necessary to supply fat for successful broiling and improvement of flavor. It is difficult to add fat to the fish while it is broiling, so, as a rule, the fat is spread over the surface of the fish after it has been removed from the broiler. The fat may consist of broiled strips of bacon or salt pork, or it may be merely melted butter or other fat.

BROILED FISH -2

Bluefish, young cod, mackerel, salmon, large trout, and all other fish, when they weigh between half a pound and four pounds, are nice for broiling. When smaller or larger they are not so good. Always use a double broiler, which, before putting the fish into it, rub with butter. This prevents sticking. The thickness of the fish will have to be the guide in broiling.

A bluefish weighing four pounds will take from twenty minutes to half an hour to cook. Many cooks brown the fish handsomely over the coals and then put it into the oven to finish broiling. Where the fish is very thick, this is a good plan. If the fish is taken from the broiler to be put into the oven, it should be slipped on to a tin sheet, that it may slide easily into the platter at serving time; for nothing so mars a dish of fish as to have it come to the table broken. In broiling, the inside should be exposed to the fire first, and then the skin.

Great care must be taken that the skin does not burn. Mackerel will broil in from twelve to twenty minutes, young cod (also called scrod) in from twenty to thirty minutes, bluefish in from twenty to thirty minutes, salmon, in from twelve to twenty minutes, and whitefish, bass, mullet, etc., in about eighteen minutes. All kinds of broiled fish can be served with a seasoning of salt, pepper and butter, or with any fish sauces. Always, when possible, garnish with parsley or something else green.

BROILED SCROD WITH POTATO BORDER.

Young cod that is split down the back and that has had the backbone removed with the exception of a small portion near the tail is known as scrod. Such fish is nearly always broiled, it may be served plain, but it is much more attractive when potatoes are combined with it in the form of an artistic border.

To prepare this dish, broil the scrod according to the directions given here, then place it on a hot platter and spread butter over it. Boil the desired number of potatoes until they are tender, and then force them through a ricer or mash them until they are perfectly fine.

Season with salt, pepper, and butter, and add sufficient milk to make a paste that is a trifle stiffer than for mashed potatoes. If desired, raw eggs may also be beaten into the potatoes to serve as a part of the moisture. Fill a pastry bag with the potatoes thus prepared and press them through a rosette tube in any desired design on the platter around the fish. Bake in a hot oven until the potatoes are thoroughly heated and are browned slightly on the top.

BROILED FRESH MACKEREL.

Probably no fish lends itself better to broiling than fresh mackerel, as the flesh of this fish is tender and contains sufficient fat to have a good flavor. To improve the flavor, however, strips of bacon are usually placed over the fish and allowed to broil with it.

Clean and skin a fresh mackerel. Place the fish thus prepared in a broiler, and broil first on one side and then on the other. When seared all over, place strips of bacon over the fish and continue to broil until it is done. Remove from the broiler, season with salt and pepper, and serve.

BROILED SHAD ROE.

The mass of eggs found in shad is known as the 'roe of shad'. Roe may be purchased separately, when it is found in the markets, or it may be procured from the fish itself. It makes a delicious dish when broiled, especially when it is rolled in fat and bread crumbs.

Wash the roe that is to be used and dry it carefully between towels. Roll it in bacon fat or melted butter and then in fine crumbs. Place in a broiler, broil until completely done on one side, turn and then broil until entirely cooked on the other side. Remove from the broiler and pour melted butter over each piece. Sprinkle with salt and pepper, and serve hot.

BROILED SALMON.

Cut the slices one inch thick, and season them with pepper and salt; butter a sheet of white paper, lay each slice on a separate piece, envelop them in it with their ends twisted; broil gently over a clear fire, and serve with anchovy or caper sauce. When higher seasoning is required, add a few chopped herbs and a little spice.

BROILED SALT SALMON

Soak salmon in tepid or cold water twenty-four hours, changing water several times, or let stand under faucet of running water. If in hurry, or desiring a very salt relish, it may do to soak a short time, having water warm, and changing, parboiling slightly. At the hour wanted, broil sharply. Season to suit taste, covering with butter. This recipe will answer for all kinds of salt fish.

BROILED HALIBUT.

Season the slices with salt and pepper, and lay them in melted butter for half an hour, having them well covered on both sides. Roll in flour, and broil for twelve minutes over a clear fire. Serve on a hot dish, garnishing with parsley and slices of lemon. The slices of halibut should be about an inch thick, and for every pound there should be three table-spoonfuls of butter.

BAKED FISH.

Good-sized fish, that is, fish weighing 4 or 5 pounds, are usually baked. When prepared by this method, fish are very satisfactory if they are spread out on a pan, flesh side up, and baked in a very hot oven with sufficient fat to flavor them well. A fish of large size, however, is especially delicious if its cavity is filled with a stuffing before it is baked.

When a fish is to be stuffed, any desired stuffing is prepared and then filled into the fish. With the cavity well filled, the edges of the fish are drawn together over the stuffing and sewed with a coarse needle and thread.

Whether the fish is stuffed or not, the same principles apply in its baking as apply in the roasting of meat; that is, the heat of a quick, hot oven sears the flesh, keeps in the juices, and prevents the loss of flavor, while that of a slow oven causes the loss of much of the flavor and moisture and produces a less tender dish. Often, in the baking of fish, it is necessary to add fat. This may be done by putting fat of some kind into the pan with the fish.

BAKED HADDOCK.

As haddock is a good-sized fish, it is an especially suitable one for baking. However, it is a dry fish, so fat should be added to it to improve its flavor. When haddock is to be baked, select a 4 or 5-pound fish, clean it thoroughly, boning it if desired, and sprinkle it inside and out with salt. Fill the cavity with any desired stuffing and sew up. Place in a dripping pan, and add some fat or place several slices of high fat meat around it. Bake in a hot oven for about 1 hour. After it has been in the oven for about 15 minutes, baste with the fat that will be found in the bottom of the pan and continue to baste every 10 minutes until the fish is done. Remove from the pan to a platter, garnish with parsley and slices of meat, and serve with any desired sauce.

BAKED HALIBUT.

Because of its size, halibut is cut into slices and sold in the form of steaks. Halibut slices are often sautéed, but they make a delicious dish when baked with tomatoes and flavored with onion, lemon, and bay leaf.

2 c. tomatoes

Few slices onion

1 bay leaf

1 tsp. salt

1/8 tsp. pepper

2 thin slices bacon

1 Tb. flour

2 lb. halibut steak

Heat the tomatoes, onion, and bay leaf in water. Add the salt and pepper and cook for a few minutes. Cut the bacon into small squares, try it out in a pan, and into this fat stir the flour. Pour this into the hot mixture, remove the bay leaf, and cook until the mixture thickens. Put the steaks into a baking dish, pour the sauce over them, and bake in a slow oven for about 45 minutes. Remove with the sauce to a hot platter and serve.

BAKED SALMON TROUT.

This deliciously flavored game-fish is baked precisely as shad or white fish, but should be accompanied with cream gravy to make it perfect. It should be baked slowly, basting often with butter and water. When done have ready in a saucepan a cup of cream, diluted with a few spoonfuls of hot water, for fear it might clot in heating, in which have been stirred cautiously two tablespoonfuls of melted butter, a scant tablespoonful of flour, and a little chopped parsley. Heat this in a vessel set within another of boiling water, add the gravy from the dripping-pan, boil up once to thicken, and when the trout is laid on a suitable hot dish, pour this sauce around it. Garnish with sprigs of parsley.

BAKED SALMON WHOLE

Having cleaned a small or moderate sized salmon, season it with salt, pepper, and powdered mace rubbed on it both outside and in. Skewer it with the tail turned round and put to the mouth. Lay it on a stand or trivet in a deep dish or pan, and stick it over with bits of butter rolled in flour. Put it into the oven, and baste it occasionally, while baking, with its own drippings. Garnish it with horseradish and sprigs of curled parsley, laid alternately round the edge of the dish; and send to table with it a small tureen of lobster sauce.

BAKED BLUEFISH

Take 2 lb Bluefish fillets, 1/2 c. Milk, 1 c. Bread crumbs, 1/4 lb Butter, 2 tb Lemon juice, 1/2 c Seafood seasoning, Salt and pepper to taste. Preheat the oven to 450°. Dip fish in milk; sprinkle lightly with salt and pepper. Coat fish with the bread crumbs. Place 1/2 table-spoon butter on each fillet; sprinkle with lemon juice and fish seasoning. Place fish in well buttered baking pan. Bake for ten to fifteen minutes.

BAKED FILLETS OF WHITEFISH.

When whitefish of medium size can be secured, it is very often stuffed and baked whole, but variety can be had by cutting it into fillets before baking it. Besides producing a delicious dish, this method of preparation eliminates carving at the table, for the pieces can be cut the desired size for serving.

Prepare fillets of whitefish according to the directions given for filleting fish. Sprinkle each one with salt and pepper, and dip it first into beaten egg and then into bread crumbs. Brown some butter in a pan, place the fish into it, and set the pan in a hot oven. Bake until the fillets are a light brown, or about 30 minutes. Remove to a hot dish, garnish with parsley and serve with any desired sauce.

BAKED FINNAN HADDIE.

When haddock is cured by smoking, it is known as 'finnan haddie'. As fish of this kind has considerable thick flesh, it is very good for baking. Other methods of cookery may, of course, be applied to it, but none is more satisfactory than baking. To bake a finnan haddie, wash it in warm water and put it to soak in fresh warm water. After it has soaked for 1/2 hour, allow it to come gradually to nearly the boiling point and then pour off the water. Place the fish in a baking pan, add a piece of butter, sprinkle with pepper, and pour a little water over it. Bake in a hot oven until it is nicely browned. Serve hot.

BAKED ROCK FISH.

Rub the fish with salt, black pepper, and a dust of cayenne, inside and out; prepare a stuffing of bread and butter, seasoned with pepper, salt, parsley and thyme; mix an egg in it, fill the fish with this, and sew it up or tie a string round it; put it in a deep pan, or oval oven and bake it as you would a fowl. To a large fish add half a pint of water; you can add more for the gravy if necessary; dust flour over and baste it with butter. Any other fresh fish can be baked in the same way. A large one will bake slowly in an hour and a half, small ones in half an hour.

CASSEROLE OF FISH

Cook 1 cupful of rice or barley. Measure the ingredients given in Salmon Timbale or Loaf, using salmon or any kind of canned or cooked fish, and prepare a fish loaf. Let the cereal cool slightly after cooking. Then line a baking dish or a mold with about three fourths of the cooked rice or barley, pressing it in the dish firmly with a spoon. Put the fish mixture in the cavity and cover it with the remainder of the cereal. Steam the food 30 to 45 minutes. Turn from the mold and serve hot with White Sauce as directed for Salmon Timbale.

CREAMED CODFISH.

Since codfish is a rather dry fish, containing little fat, it is usually combined with some other food to make it more appetizing. In the case of creamed codfish, the cream sauce supplies the food substances in which the fish is lacking and at the same time provides a very palatable dish. When codfish is prepared in this way, boiled potatoes are usually served with it.

To make creamed codfish, freshen the required amount of codfish by pouring lukewarm water over it. Shred the fish by breaking it into small pieces with the fingers. Pour off the water, add fresh warm water, and allow the fish to stand until it is not too salty. When it is sufficiently freshened, drain off all the water. Melt a little butter in a frying pan, add the fish, and sauté until slightly browned. Make a medium white sauce and pour it over the codfish. Serve hot with boiled potatoes.

CREAMED FINNAN HADDIE.

The flavor of finnan haddie is such that this fish becomes very appetizing when prepared with a cream sauce. If, after combining the sauce with the fish, the fish is baked in the oven, an especially palatable dish is the result. To prepare creamed finnan haddie, freshen the fish and shred it into small pieces. Then measure the fish, put it into a baking dish, and pour an equal amount of white sauce over it. Sprinkle generously with crumbs and bake in a hot oven until the crumbs are browned. Serve hot.

CREAMED TUNA FISH.

Combining canned tuna fish with a cream sauce and serving it over toast makes a dish that is both delicate and palatable one that will prove very satisfactory when something to take the place of meat in a light meal is desired.

3 Tb. butter

3 Tb. flour

1/2 tsp. salt

1/8 tsp. pepper

1/8 tsp. paprika

1-1/2 c. hot milk

1-1/2 c. tuna fish

1 egg

Melt the butter in a saucepan and add the flour, salt, pepper, and paprika. Stir well, pour in the milk, and when this has thickened add the tuna fish. Allow this to heat thoroughly in the sauce. Just before serving, add the slightly beaten egg and cook until this has thickened.

Pour over toast and serve. Sufficient to Serve Six.

CREAMED SALMON WITH RICE.

A creamed protein dish is always more satisfactory if it is served on some other food, particularly one high in carbohydrate. When this is done, a better balanced dish is the result. Creamed salmon and rice make a very nutritious and appetizing combination.

1 c. salmon

1 c. medium white sauce

Steamed rice

Break the salmon into moderately small pieces and carefully fold these into the hot white sauce. Serve this on a mound of hot steamed rice.

CREAMED FISH IN POTATO NEST.

Fish may also be combined with mashed potato to produce a most appetizing dish. Line a baking dish with hot mashed potato, leaving a good-sized hollow in the center. Into this pour creamed fish made by mixing equal proportions of cold fish and white sauce. Season well with salt and pepper, sprinkle with crumbs, and dot the top with butter. Bake until the crumbs are brown. Serve hot.

CODFISH BALLS.

One pound codfish; one and a half pound potatoes; one quarter pound butter; two eggs. Boil the fish slowly, then pound with a potato masher until very fine; add the potatoes mashed and hot; next add butter and one-half cup milk and the two eggs. Mix thoroughly, form into balls, and fry in hot fat.

CODFISH SOUP

Take one-half pound of salt codfish that has been soaked, cut it up into squares, but not small. Prepare in a saucepan four tablespoons of good olive-oil, and one small onion cut into pieces. Cook the onion in the oil over a slow fire, without allowing the onion to become colored, and then add a small bunch of parsley stems, a small piece of celery, a bay-leaf, and a small sprig of thyme. Cool for a few moments, then add two tomatoes, skinned and with the seeds removed, and cut into slices, two tablespoons of dry white wine, and one medium-sized potato, peeled and cut into slices, and, lastly, one cup of water.

When the potato is half cooked, add the codfish, then one-half tablespoon more of olive-oil. Remove the parsley stems, and put in instead one-half tablespoon of chopped-up parsley; add a good pinch of pepper, and some salt, if needed. When the vegetables are thoroughly cooked pour the soup over pieces of toasted or fried bread, and serve.

ABOUT THE AUTHOR

Anna Reed loves cooking. She is from a family of great cook. Anna somehow created great recipes that are healthy yet still very enticing and scrumptious to eat.

This started when Anna has a family of her own. Not Ann wants to feed her family but she wants to make sure that she is preparing the right healthy meal. She then became nutritionist and health buff.

www.ingramcontent.com/pod-product-compliance
Lightning Source LLC
Chambersburg PA
CBHW070034260726
48658CB00002B/628